漫画中药故事系列
Chinese Medicines in Cartoon Series

名医药传
（汉英对照）

Tales of Doctors and TCM
(Chinese-English)

U0287860

杨柏灿　**主编**
Edited by Yang Baican

杨熠文　晋　永　鲍思思　祝建龙　◎**文/译**
Paperwork by Yang Yiwen, Jin Yong, Bao Sisi, Zhu Jianlong

孔珏莹　夏瑜桢　金潇逸　◎**绘**
Brushwork by Kong Jueying, Xia Yuzhen, Jin Xiaoyi

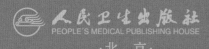

人民卫生出版社
PEOPLE'S MEDICAL PUBLISHING HOUSE
·北 京·

图书在版编目（CIP）数据

名医药传：汉英对照 / 杨柏灿主编 . —北京：人民卫生出版社，2021.3

（漫画中药故事系列）

ISBN 978-7-117-31329-2

I. ①名… II. ①杨… III. ①中药材 – 普及读物 – 汉、英 IV. ①R282-49

中国版本图书馆 CIP 数据核字（2021）第 037644 号

人卫智网	www.ipmph.com	医学教育、学术、考试、健康，
		购书智慧智能综合服务平台
人卫官网	www.pmph.com	人卫官方资讯发布平台

漫画中药故事系列——名医药传（汉英对照）
Manhua Zhongyao Gushi Xilie——Mingyi Yaozhuan（Han-Ying Duizhao）

主　　编：杨柏灿
出版发行：人民卫生出版社（中继线 010-59780011）
地　　址：北京市朝阳区潘家园南里 19 号
邮　　编：100021
E - mail：pmph @ pmph.com
购书热线：010-59787592　010-59787584　010-65264830
印　　刷：北京顶佳世纪印刷有限公司
经　　销：新华书店
开　　本：889×1194　1/24　印张：3.5
字　　数：102 千字
版　　次：2021 年 3 月第 1 版
印　　次：2021 年 4 月第 1 次印刷
标准书号：ISBN 978-7-117-31329-2
定　　价：50.00 元

打击盗版举报电话：010-59787491　E-mail：WQ @ pmph.com
质量问题联系电话：010-59787234　E-mail：zhiliang @ pmph.com

序言

由上海中医药大学杨柏灿教授主编的《漫画中药故事系列》由人民卫生出版社出版了。这也是杨教授十年来从事中医药文化研究、作品创作和开展中医药文化普及工作的又一力作。

中医药是中国优秀传统文化的代表，凝聚着深邃的中国古代哲学智慧和科学文明的精髓。在抗击新冠肺炎疫情中，中医药发挥了突出的作用，引起世人的高度关注。国家的重视、社会的认同和关注，使中医药的发展迎来了前所未有的大好时机。抓住这一千载难逢的契机，做好中医药的传承与创新、推广与普及工作，是每一位中医药工作者义不容辞的责任。

做好中医药的传承、创新与弘扬，首先重在传承，只有真正做好传承，将中医药的精气神传承下来，才有可能不断创新、发展、弘扬。要做好中医药的传承，除了专业院校的教学以及师承以外，在全社会开展中医药知识的普及推广是一项十分重要的工作，特别是重视"从娃娃抓起"，从小就让我们的孩子沐浴中医药知识的阳光雨露，领略中医药世界的奥秘，感受中国传统文化的伟大，树立文化自信，使之入心入脑，有助于增强孩子们的民族自豪感，激发爱国情怀。

Foreword

Chinese Medicines in Cartoon Series compiled by Professor Yang Baican from Shanghai University of Traditional Chinese Medicine (SHTCM) is published by People's Medical Publishing House. It is a masterpiece by Professor Yang after his 10-year study on, writing about and popularization of Chinese medicine culture.

Traditional Chinese medicine (TCM) is representative of traditional Chinese culture, where lies the wisdom of ancient Chinese philosophy and the essence of scientific civilization. In the fight against COVID-19 epidemic, TCM has been playing an important role and attracts a lot of attention. Valued by the nation and accepted and followed with interest by the society, TCM has an unprecedented opportunity for development. It is a duty for every TCM worker to seize this opportunity and perform well in inheritance, innovation, promotion and popularization of TCM.

To inherit, innovate and carry forward TCM, inheritance is the first and foremost. TCM can be innovated, developed and carried forward only when it is inherited properly with its essence handed down. For inheritance of TCM, besides teachings in professional schools and from a master to his/her apprentices, it is important to popularize TCM knowledge in the whole society, with focus on "Starts with children". Let our children bathe in the sunshine of TCM knowledge, get to know the mystery of TCM and feel the magnificence of traditional Chinese culture, so that they can have cultural confidence, which helps enhance their sense of national pride and inspire their love for the country.

近年来，一些有识之士已开展了卓有成效的"中医药走进中小学"的工作，受到了广泛的关注和认同。伴随着国家综合实力的增强，我国国际社会地位的提升，中医药的国际影响力也日益扩大。重视中医药走向国际，弘扬中国传统文化，不但有利于提升我国文化软实力，而且也有益于中医药为全人类造福。

杨柏灿教授是上海中医药大学从事中药学教学的教师。他在完成中医药的医、教、研工作之余，十年来致力于中医药知识的推广与普及工作，在国内最早开设了中药慕课课程《走近中药》《杏林探宝——带你走进中药》《杏林探宝——认知中药》《中药学》《中药知多少》以及微视频《中药知识——走进中小学》。其中《杏林探宝——认知中药》上线美国 Coursera 平台，受众人群遍及 80 余个国家和地区，学习人数达 10 余万人次。同时，杨教授笔耕不辍，六年来先后出版了中医药通识读本《药缘文化——中药与文化的交融》《药名文化——中药与文化的交融》，连续三年出版了《本草光阴——中药养生文化日历》，在社会上产生一定的影响。

In recent years, men of sight have carried out projects of "Introducing TCM into middle and primary schools", which is widely concerned and approved. With enhancement of the overall national strength and the elevated status of China in the international community, TCM has an increasingly large international influence. Paying attention to international communication of TCM and carrying forward traditional Chinese culture can not only strengthen the cultural soft power of China, but also bring benefit for all mankind.

The author is a professor in Chinese medicines in SHTCM. After finishing his work as a doctor, teacher and researcher in TCM, he has been dedicated to promotion and popularization of TCM knowledge for nearly a decade. He is the first to provide MOOCs on Chinese medicines in China, including *Get Closer to Chinese Medicines*, *Hunt for Treasure in Apricot Grove — Bring You Closer to Chinese Medicines*, *Hunt for Treasure in Apricot Grove — Get to Know Chinese Medicines*, *Traditional Chinese Pharmacology* and *What Do You Know About Chinese Medicines*, as well as a micro video of *Knowledge about Chinese Medicines — Introduced into Middle and Primary Schools*. Among them, *Hunt for Treasure in Apricot Grove — Get to Know Chinese Medicines* is available online on Coursera, with audience from more than 80 countries and regions and learned by over 100,000 person-time. At the same time, Professor Yang has been writing continuously. In recent six years, he has published books on TCM including *Medicine Culture—Blending of Chinese Medicines and Culture* and *Medicine Name Culture—Blending of Chinese Medicines and Culture* and has published *Time and Chinese Materia Medica—Health Culture Calendar with Chinese Medicines*, which has a certain social impact.

《漫画中药故事系列》突破了目前市面上单纯以文字讲中药故事，或是将中药故事与中药知识相割离的作品形式，遍查古籍，选取有史实依据、民众知晓度高、具有深厚中国传统文化底蕴的中药故事，通过生动形象的漫画和精练朴实的语言，讲解中药故事，向世人展示中药知识与中国多元优秀传统文化的交融。读者在赏读本丛书时，不但能了解常用的中药知识，还能在不知不觉中接受中国传统文化的熏陶。本丛书的文字部分采用中英文对照的形式，益于中医药在国际上传播，同时也使中小学生在阅读漫画、接受中医药知识之余，提升英语的阅读能力。

本丛书的出版发行对于中医药的推广、普及势必有一定的促进作用，期待杨柏灿教授团队能不断有新的作品问世。

Chinese Medicines in Cartoon Series gets rid of the layout of telling stories about Chinese medicines in words alone or separating the stories from the knowledge. The author has consulted ancient books and selected the stories that are based on historical facts, well known among people and deeply rooted in traditional Chinese culture. The stories about Chinese medicines are told through vivid cartoons and in simple language. They show the world the blending of knowledge about Chinese medicines with traditional Chinese culture, so that the reader can not only know about Chinese medicines, but also feel the charm of traditional Chinese culture. The text part of the series of books is in both Chinese and English to promote international spread of TCM, and additionally, the students in middle and primary schools can have their English reading ability improved while reading the cartoons and learning about Chinese medicines.

Publishing and distribution of this series of books will surely give an impetus to the promotion and popularization of TCM and I look forward to more works by the team led by Professor Yang Baican.

上海市卫生健康委员会副主任
上海市中医药管理局副局长
上海中医药学会会长
原上海中医药大学副校长

胡鸿毅

2020 年 9 月

Deputy director, Shanghai Municipal Health Commission

Deputy director, Shanghai Municipal Administrator of Traditional Chinese Medicine

President, Shanghai Association of Traditional Chinese Medicine

Former vice-president, Shanghai University of Traditional Chinese Medicine

Hu Hongyi

Sep, 2020

神農尝草五千載
名醫良藥百世彰
醫者雖無通天術
却以妙手起沉痾
博觀厚積仁心在
奉草精神共承傳

前言

Preface

随着我国综合实力的不断提高和国际地位的日益提升，文化软实力建设、树立文化自信，已成为国家的发展战略。习近平总书记指出"中医药学凝聚着深邃的哲学智慧和中华民族几千年的健康养生理念及其实践经验，是中国古代科学的瑰宝，也是打开中华文明宝库的钥匙"，高屋建瓴地概括了中医药在传统文化中具有不可替代的地位及其所具有的鲜明的文化特征。

With its increasing comprehensive strength and growing status in the world, China's cultural soft power along with cultural confidence turns to renascent tendency. Chinese President Xi Jinping, once claimed that "Traditional Chinese medical theory is the gem of ancient Chinese science and philosophy, and also a key to the treasure of Chinese civilization", reconfirming the irreplaceable position and distinct feature of traditional Chinese medicine (TCM) in our culture.

《漫画中药故事系列》以历史悠久、扎根于中华大地、深植于大众心灵的中药为切入点，通过具有史料记载、民间知晓度高的典故传说，采用形象生动的漫画形式，传播中药知识，弘扬传统文化。丛书共分四册，既可独立成书又前后互为关联。

Chinese Medicines in Cartoon Series aims at spreading knowledge of TCM and promoting our national culture. The series takes the well-known herbs as entry, tells fact-based tales and illustrates stories with pictures in comic format. The series includes four books, each being a sub-topic of TCM.

第一册《名医药传》：从中药雅称、药物应用、功效发现，介绍家喻户晓的名医名家治疗顽苛痼疾、疑难杂症的故事。

Book I *Tales of Doctors and TCM*: stories about miscellaneous and critical cases, mainly from the aspects of herbs' poetic names and efficacy.

第二册《君药传奇》：从药名来历、药物应用等方面，介绍中药与古代君王间的趣闻典故以及民间医药高手不畏权贵、巧用中药的故事。

Book II *Tales of Emperors and TCM*: stories about emperors and herbs, mainly from the aspects of herbs' naming and efficacy.

第三册《品读中药》：从汤羹、酒与豆腐发明的故事，介绍中药与饮食文化的渊源，体现药食同源的特性；通过益母草、王不留行、远志等中药名称来历的典故，体现中药药名的文化内涵。

第四册《智用中药》：从药物生长环境、采摘时节、药用部位、应用方式等对药效的影响，体现古今医药学家认识自然、应用自然的智慧。

随着国家对中医药工作日益重视以及在这次抗击新冠肺炎疫情中，中医药不可或缺的作用，重视做好中医药的传承、创新及推广已成为全社会的共识。特别是近年来，越来越多人意识到，要做好中医药的传承应该从小抓起，要重视中医药走进中小学的工作。正是在这样的大背景下，本团队经过3年多的努力，在人民卫生出版社的大力支持下，完成了以传播中药知识、弘扬传统文化为宗旨的漫画中药故事系列丛书。期望本丛书的出版发行，能有益于中医药知识和传统文化的传播。

Book Ⅲ *Tales of Food and TCM*: stories about herbs and diet through the invention of soup, wine and tofu; stories about herbs and its name origin through the naming of motherwort, polygala, etc.

Book Ⅳ *Tales of Creative Use and TCM*: stories about herbs and efficacy, mainly from the aspects of herbs' living environment, growing seasons, plant parts and application.

With the increasing emphasis on the traditional Chinese medical theory and its indispensable role in the combat against COVID-19, the whole society has reached the consensus that the traditional Chinese medical theory should be inherited, innovated as well as promoted. In recent years, more and more people have realized that the inheritance of TCM should be cultivated since childhood and that TCM should be introduced into elementary education stage. Thanks to People's Medical Publishing House, our team, after more than three years' constant efforts, has completed this series of comic books on TCM. We are hoping that Chinese medicine and traditional Chinese culture can be promoted after its publication.

考虑到中西方文化背景的不同，在英语翻译上侧重于意译，而非直译，部分内容及标题中英文有所不同，须结合具体故事情节予以理解。

本丛书适用于广大中医药爱好者，特别是中小学生。同时，本丛书中英对照的形式也有助于在国际上传播、宣传中医药知识和中国传统文化，推动中医药国际化。

《漫画中药故事系列》丛书编委会

2020 年 7 月 25 日

Owning to the cultural differences between the East and the West, some parts of the stories have been translated sense-for-sense instead word-for-word.

This series of books is written for Chinese medicine enthusiasts, especially primary and middle school students. Meanwhile, in the form of both Chinese and English, it helps to spread Chinese medicine knowledge and culture so as to promote its internationalization.

Editorial Committee

July 25, 2020

目录
CATALOG

第一部分
以药寓医传古今

在西医传入中国以前，并没有"中医"这个名字，而是有着其他独特且赋有内涵的称谓，其中也不乏与中药名称相关者。

Part I
The Elegant Name of Traditional Chinese Medicine

Before the introduction of Western medicine, there was no such name as "traditional Chinese medicine" in China. However, there were other unique and connotative terms instead, many of which were related to some specific Chinese herbs.

神农尝百草
Chinese Herbal Medicine and Shennong

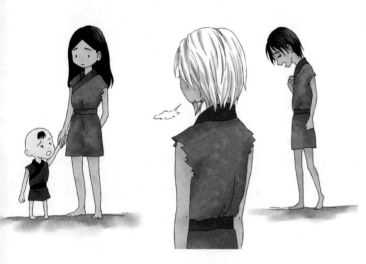

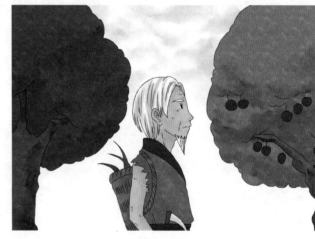

传说上古时期，原始先民常常过着茹毛饮血，食不果腹的生活。族人的疾苦，作为氏族首领的神农，看在眼里，急在心里。

Legend has it that in ancient times, our primitive ancestors often lived a life of eating raw meat and drinking blood, having far inadequate food supplies. Seeing all the sufferings, Shennong, the clan leader, felt deeply sympathetic to all the sufferings his clansmen were bearing.

为了改善族人的生活，神农走上了寻食采药的旅途。每遇一种植物，他便亲自品尝并记录下它的味道和食后反应，并以此为同族居民果腹治病。

In order to improve the lives of his clansmen, Shennong embarked on a journey to find food and medicine. Each time he found a plant, he would personally taste it, test it, ascertain its medicinal value, and then use it to help relieve his people of their afflictions and sufferings.

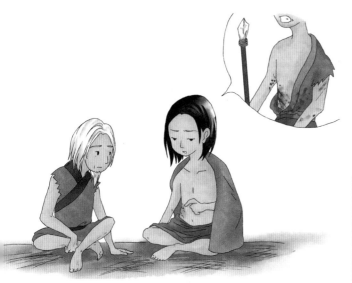

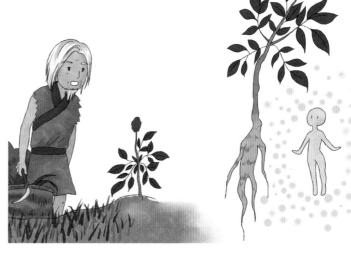

一日，神农所在氏族的族人，在一次狩猎中不慎受伤，待他伤口痊愈后，却一直虚弱无力。

One day, one of his clansmen got hurt in a hunting accident. He, though recovered from his wounds, still remained weak.

在一次采药中，神农发现有一种植物旁边几乎无杂草树木，感觉甚是奇怪，于是便将其挖出，发现其根竟然如同人形。

During his herb collection, Shennong caught sight of a plant with almost no weeds nearby, which was quite unusual. Therefore, he dug it out and surprisingly found that the shape of its root resembled that of a human.

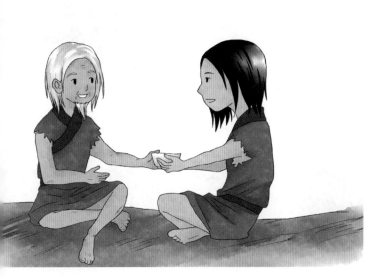

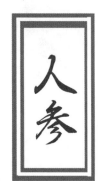

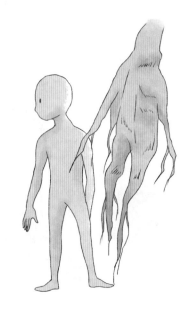

联想到它的生长环境，神农意识到这种植物必然
积聚自然之精华，于是便将其给那位受伤后虚弱
的族人试服，果不其然该族人恢复了元气。

Associating with the environment in which it
grew, Shennong realized that the plant must have
accumulated the essence of nature, so he took it
and gave it to the patient and, sure enough, the man
restored his energy and vitality.

这味药物便是如今闻名的"人参"，恰因其形似
"人"而得名。

This herb is now known as "Ren Shen" (Ginseng),
which is named for its resemblance to human beings
("Ren" in Chinese).

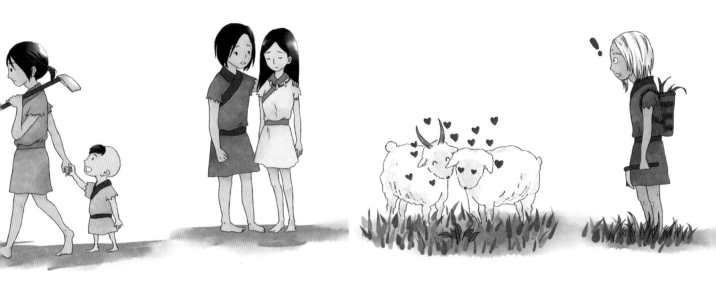

神农所在族群总有许多人一直苦于无后代，族群的繁衍与发展受到很大的限制，神农为此感到担忧。

Many of Shennong's clansmen had fertility problems, resulting in the restriction of the clan development. That worried Shennong a lot.

神农在上山寻药过程中，发现每当羊在啃食一种草后，羊和羊总是不断交合。

In the process of searching for medicine on the mountain, Shennong found that sheep always copulated constantly after they had eaten a certain kind of plant.

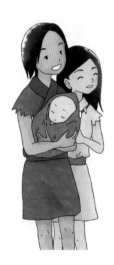
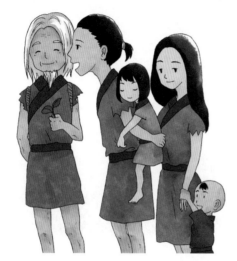
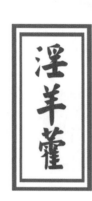
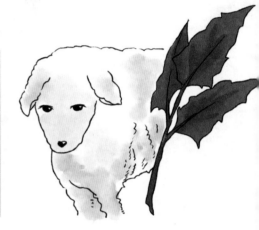

于是他感觉这味药可能有促进繁衍的作用，便将其采来给族人服下。果然，之后几年族群的人丁日渐兴旺了起来。

Instinctively, Shennong felt that this plant might help fertility, so he collected it and brought it back to his clansmen. As was expected, the population of the ethnic group began to boom over the next few years.

由于这味药因羊发现，羊食后不断交合，便将其命名为"淫羊藿"。

As the discovery of this herb was sheep-associated—sheep continue to copulate after eating, accordingly, it is named "Yin Yang ("Sheep" in English) Huo" (Herba Epimedii).

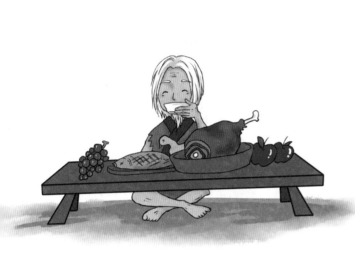

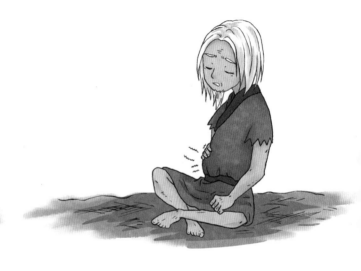

族群在过去的一年迎来了大丰收，神农与族人一起举办了一场庆功宴，在宴会上神农吃了不少大鱼大肉。

Once the clan had a great harvest. Shennong and his people celebrated it with a banquet. At the banquet, there was abundant fish and meat, which Shennong took in a lot.

可之后几天，神农却出现了便秘，好几天都没有排便，腹部胀痛甚是痛苦。

However, in the next few days, Shennong became constipated and had no defecation for several days. He felt absolutely bloated.

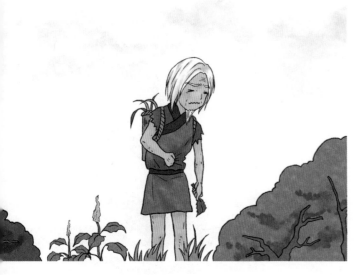

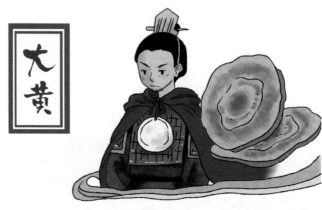

神农想起以前在采药时吃过的一种草具有通便的作用，于是就采来服下，不久便觉腹痛难忍，不多时即解下大便，人也舒畅了许多。

这味药其色黄而作用强，故将其命名为"大黄"。

Shennong recalled that in the past, a kind of herb had the effect of defecation, so he picked it and took it. Soon he felt unbearable abdominal pain and immediately released his stools. And naturally he felt a lot carefree.

This herb is yellow ("Huang" in Chinese) in color and strong ("Da" in Chinese) in effect, so it is called "Da Huang" (Radix et Rhizoma Rhei).

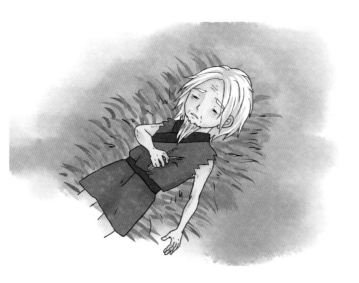

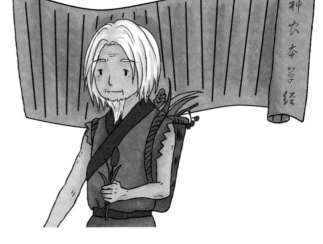

不幸的是，在一次采药过程中，神农因误尝了剧毒的断肠草而离世。

神农便是后世传颂的炎帝，为了纪念他对人类发展的贡献，中华民族常常以炎黄子孙自称。而后世医家更是托神农之名编撰本草学专著《神农本草经》。

Unfortunately, in the course of a medicinal collection, Shennong died from mistakenly taking *Gelsemium elegans*, a highly toxic yellow-flowered shrub known as heartbreak grass.

Shennong, also known as the Yan Emperor, was eulogized everywhere in later generations. In order to commemorate his outstanding contribution to human development, the Chinese people often call themselves "descendants of the Yan and Huang Emperors". Moreover, later generations of medical experts began to compile the pharmacopoeia *Shennong's Herbal Classic* in the name of Shennong.

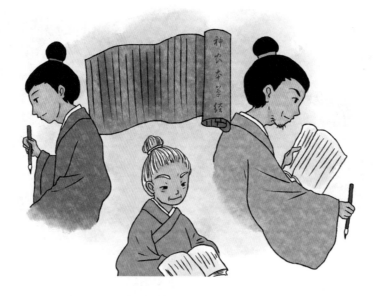

《神农本草经》

Shennong's Herbal Classic

《神农本草经》

由于中药中多为植物药，故中药在古时被称为本草，后世的中药典籍也常以"本草"命名，如《神农本草经》《本草纲目》等。其中《神农本草经》中共载药 365 味，以三品分类法将其分为上（无毒，能延年益寿）、中（无毒有毒，既能补养又能祛邪）、下（多毒，祛邪为主）三品，它奠定了中药理论的基础。不论神农尝百草的故事只是一个传说还是上古先人尝药发现的总汇，不可否认的是：中医药有如今的发展与成就，是建立在历朝历代如神农氏般的医者、医家反复的实践与总结基础上的。

Shennong's Herbal Classic

Since most of the traditional Chinese medicines are natural plants, they were called "Ben ('Source' in English) Cao ('Plant' in English)" in ancient times, and later Chinese medicine classics were also named after "Ben Cao", such as "Shennong Ben Cao Jing" (*Shennong's Herbal Classic*) and "Ben Cao Gang Mu" (*Compendium of Materia Medica*). The Chinese literary work *Shennong's Herbal Classic* is said to have classified 365 species of medicines in three categories: superior (non-poisonous and rejuvenating), medium (having some toxicity based on the dosage and exerting tonic effects) and inferior (poisonous but able to quickly reduce fever, cure indigestion, etc.), which later lay the foundation of herbalogical studies in China for thousands of years. Whether the story of Shennong is just a legend or his book a compilation of discoveries of numerous ancient ancestors tasting herbs, it is undeniable that the development and achievements of traditional Chinese medicine nowadays are based on repeated practice and summary of doctors like Shennong in successive dynasties.

杏林春暖
Apricot and Dong Feng

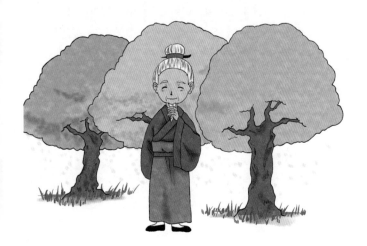

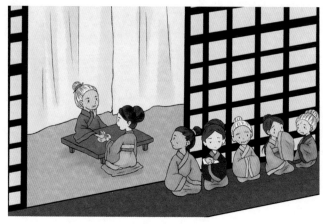

董奉为东汉末年一位杰出的医家，与张仲景、华佗，并称"建安三神医"。董奉曾留下一段脍炙人口并被后世誉为医家典范的杏林佳话。

Dong Feng was an outstanding doctor in the late Eastern Han Dynasty. Along with fellow healers Zhang Zhongjing and Hua Tuo, he was one of the "Three Divine Doctors of Jian'an Period". Many legends surround the life and work of this enlightened doctor, one of which is the famous "apricot forest" story.

董奉为福建长乐人，其精通医理，医术出众，并长年在庐山行医。不管病人有什么疑难杂症，在他面前总能够药到病除，因而前来求医问药的患者总是络绎不绝。

Dong Feng was a native of Changle County, Fujian Province. He was proficient in medical science and outstanding in medical skills, and had been practicing medicine for many years in Mount Lu in central China. No matter what difficult and complicated disease the patient had, he could always get rid of it with Dong's treatment. Therefore, there was always a constant stream of patients coming to seek medical advice from him.

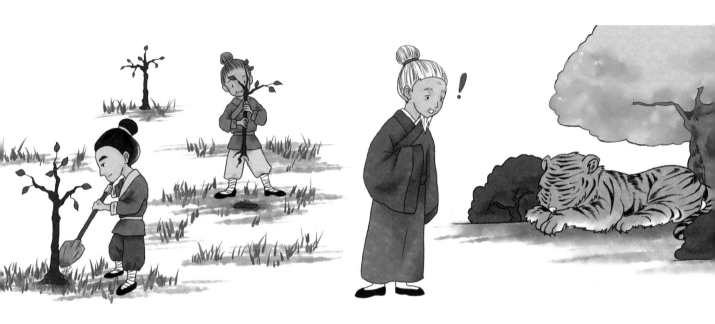

董奉为人治病从不收取任何费用。但他却有一个
要求，经他治愈的患者要在他门前种杏树。病情
轻的栽一棵，病情重的栽五棵。很快，在他诊所
周围有了一大片茂密的杏林。

Dong Feng never charged his patients any fees for a
consultation. Instead, he asked those who were cured
of serious diseases to plant five apricot trees, and those
he cured of minor ailments to plant a single apricot
tree. Very soon, there grew a dense apricot forest
around his clinic.

一日，董奉听说有一只老虎趴在他家门前，于是
便出门查看，发现那只老虎病恹恹的，表情十分
痛苦。董奉本能地感觉到这只老虎生病了。

One day, Dong Feng heard that there was a tiger lying
in front of his door. So he went out to check. Seeing the
tiger was weak and painful, Dong Feng knew for sure
that it was sick.

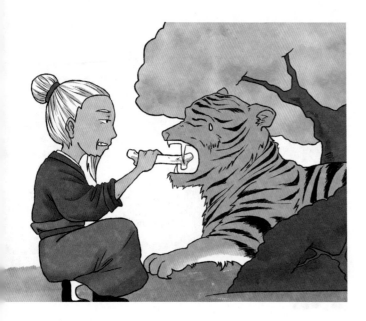

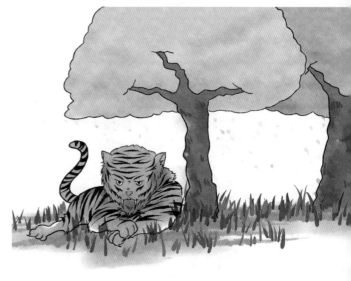

虽然心中有着些许害怕和顾虑，但医者的仁心还是让董奉决定上前诊治，这时老虎张开了嘴，董奉发现老虎喉咙中卡了一块骨头，便将虎口内的骨头取了出来，老虎的病也就好了。

Frightened as he was, Dong Feng decided to examine the tiger and give it a treatment. It was when the tiger opened its mouth that Dong Feng found a bone stuck in its throat. He took out the bone, thus healing the creature.

为了感谢董奉的救命之恩，老虎就在杏林里当起了守护。董奉治愈的人成千上万，门前的杏树自然也郁郁葱葱，蔚然成林。

In order to thank Dong Feng for saving its life, the tiger acted as a guardian in the apricot forest. Tens of thousands of people were cured by Dong Feng, and the apricot trees in front of the door were naturally lush and luxuriant.

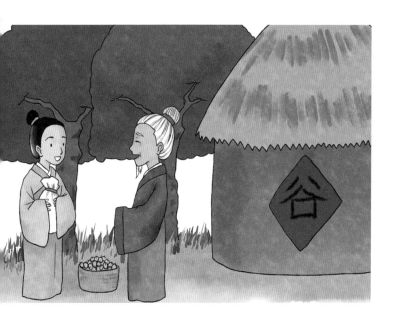

杏树成熟之际，董奉就在杏林边建起一座谷仓，以杏子交换稻谷，并将所换来的粮食用来赈救饥寒贫困的人，这便是"杏林春暖，虎守杏林"的由来。为了传扬董奉的医术医德，便尊称医界为"杏林"。

When the apricots ripened and were ready to be harvested, Dong Feng built a barn beside the apricot forest. He let people exchange rice for his apricots; the former he donated to people stricken by poverty. This is the origin of the anecdote—"Warm spring in the apricot forest, tiger guards the apricot forest". In order to respect Dong Feng's profound medical skills and his noble virtue, later medical circles are honored by being granted the title "Apricot Forest".

杏仁功效
The Efficacy of Apricot Kernel

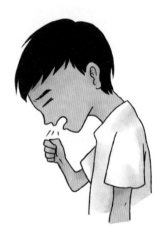

止咳平喘
Relieving cough and asthma

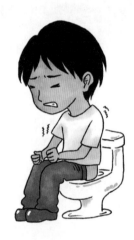

润肠通便
Relaxing bowel

功效分析

（苦）杏仁是一味十分常用的止咳平喘药。对于咳喘，无论虚实，寒热都可以用杏仁来治疗，是临床治疗咳喘的对症用药。同时杏仁为种仁类药物，其富含油脂，具有一定的润肠通便作用，临床亦可用于肠液不足、肠道干枯引起的便秘或排便困难。

Efficacy Analysis

The bitter apricot kernel is a commonly used antitussive and antiasthmatic drug. Regardless of deficiency or excess, cold and heat, it can all be treated with apricot kernel, which is the symptomatic drug for clinical treatment of cough and asthma. Meanwhile, being a kind of kernel drug, it is rich in oil and to some extent helps moisten the intestine and relieve constipation. It can also be used in clinic for constipation or defecation difficulty caused by insufficient intestinal juice or dry intestine.

橘井泉香
Tangerine and Su Dan

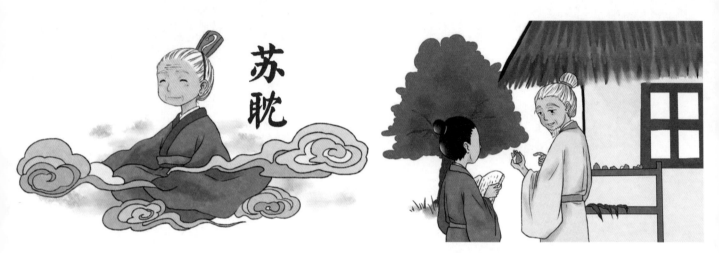

苏耽

苏耽相传是西汉时期的一位仙人，有着"苏仙公"之称。在他得道之前，他也曾是一位知名的医家。关于他的事迹，记载在葛洪的《神仙传》中。

As the legend goes, Su Dan, known as "Su Xiangong" (Daoist Immortal Su), was an immortal in the Western Han Dynasty. Before he became an immortal, he was also a famous doctor. His deeds were recorded in *The Tales of Immortals* by Ge Hong.

苏耽自幼丧父，与母亲相依为命，为人十分仁义孝顺。有一日，一位老郎中来到他居住的村子，为其孝义所感动，便将毕生所学的医术教授于他。

Losing his father at an early age, Su existed with his mother for a living. One day, a senior doctor went to his village. Moved by his filial piety, he decided to teach Su Dan all the medical skills he had ever learned.

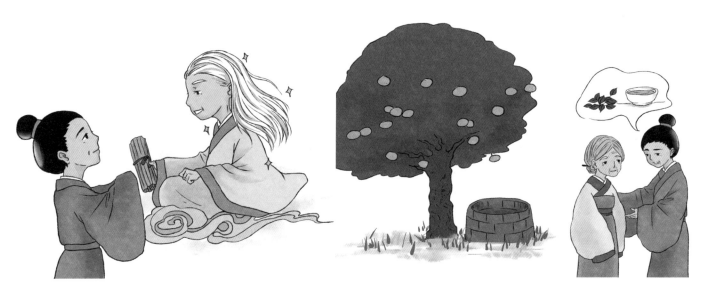

于是，苏耽便在乡里之间行医救人，受到村民的爱戴。

So, Su Dan started to practice medicine in his neighbourhood, earning him fame and respect.

一次苏耽因事需出远门，要三年后方能回家。临走之际，苏耽含泪嘱托母亲说："明年州郡恐有疫情，到时候可取庭前井水与门前的橘叶为患者治疗。"

Once Su Dan had to be away from home for three years. Before leaving, Su Dan tearfully told her mother, "There might be a plague in the county next year. In that case, you can take the well water in front of the yard and mix it with the tangerine leaves growing in the doorway. That will be the effective treatment for patients.

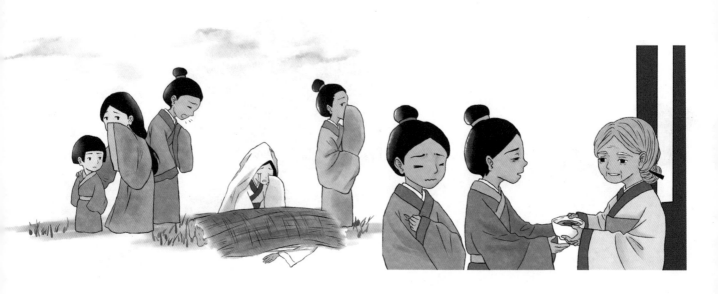

第二年，果然如苏耽所言，郴州暴发瘟疫，其来势迅猛，四处蔓延，病死无数，田间乡舍了无生气。

In the following years, just as Su Dan had predicted, the plague did break out in the Chen County, coming fiercely and spreading rapidly, causing countless deaths. In no time, the whole countryside turned out to be lifeless.

苏母便按照儿子的嘱咐，用井水煮橘叶给患者服用。

His mother, following Su's instructions, boiled the tangerine leaves with well water and gave it to the patients.

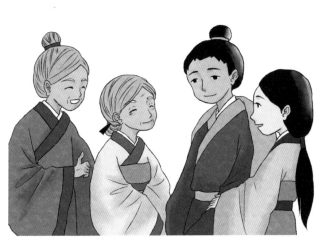

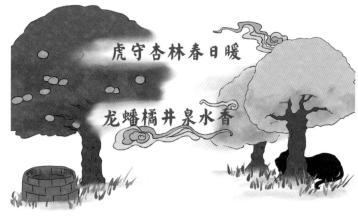

虎守杏林春日暖

龙蟠橘井泉水香

患者服后，无不痊愈，郴州的瘟疫终于得以平息，并恢复了往日的生气。

All the patients were healed. The plague in the Chen County was finally under control, and the whole area restored its previous vitality.

自此，"橘井泉香"与"杏林春暖"双璧生辉，成了中医药的象征，而董奉和苏耽也成为后世医家的典范。

Since then, "Tangerine Well with Fragrant Water" and "Warm Spring in the Apricot Forest" have become the symbols of traditional Chinese medicine. Dong Feng and Su Dan have become the models for the doctors of future generations.

橘皮功效
The Efficacy of Tangerine Peel

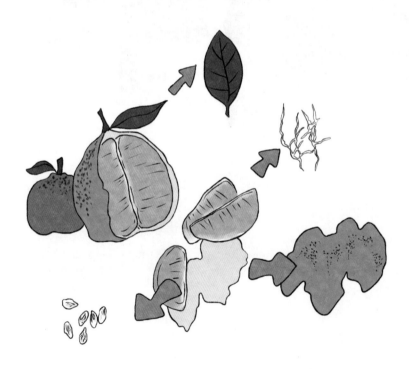

功效分析

故事中井水、橘叶是否具有如此神效无从考证。不过橘确实一身是宝，橘皮、橘络、橘核都能够作为药用。这之中最为常用的便是橘皮。橘皮又称陈皮，以陈久者为良，为代表性的理气药。功可行气燥湿，理肺健脾，主要用于脾胃不调，咳嗽多痰的治疗。

Efficacy Analysis

It is impossible to verify whether the well water and the tangerine leaves in the story have such magical effect. But the tangerine is indeed a treasure—tangerine peel, tangerine collateral, and tangerine core can be used as herbal medicine, the most commonly used of which is the tangerine peel. The tangerine peel is also called "Chen peel", "Chen" meaning "having been preserved for a long time". The longer the tangerine peel is preserved, the higher quality it will be in. The tangerine peel is the representative qi-regulating herb with the effect of activating qi and expelling the dampness, as well as regulating the lung function and invigorating the spleen. It is mainly used for the treatment of spleen and stomach disorders and cough with phlegm.

悬壶济世
Gourd and Fei Zhangfang

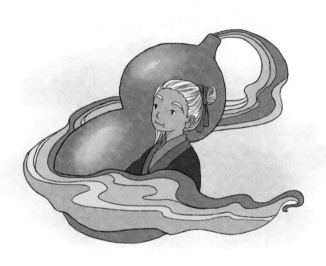

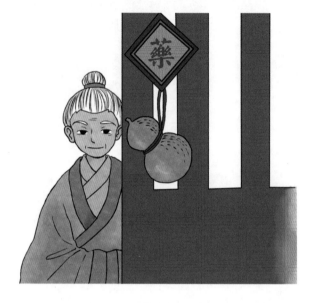

在古代医生行医的标志常用葫芦。你知道这个葫芦标志的由来吗？相传这与另一位医家费长房有关。

while in ancient times, the symbol of doctors was the gourd. Why did the gourd carry that special meaning? According to the legend, it is just because of Doctor Fei Zhangfang.

东汉时期，汝南的市场中有一位卖药的老翁，总是将一只壶挂在店铺门口，而他所卖之药甚是灵验，遂被人称为"壶公"。

In the Eastern Han Dynasty, there was an old man selling medicine in the market of Ru'nan County, Henan Province. He always hung a pot—a gourd-shaped vessel, at the door of his stall. The medicine he sold was so effective that he was honored "Grandpa Pot".

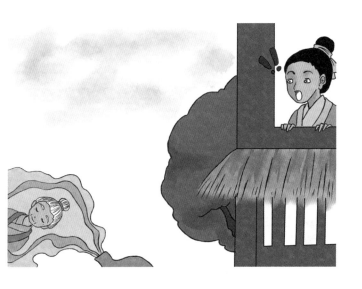

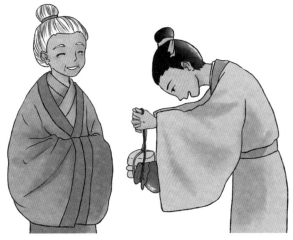

等到集市结束，街上人群散去之后，壶公便跳进壶中，而这一幕恰被费长房从楼上看到，他觉得十分奇怪，认定这卖药老翁绝非常人。

When the market closed and the crowd left, Grandpa Pot, without being noticed, soon jumped into the vessel. However, this happened to be seen by Fei Zhangfang from upstairs. He surely believed that this old man was not normal people.

第二日，他制备了酒肉，恭恭敬敬地拜见壶公。壶公在了解费长房的来意后，察其一片诚心，为可造之才，于是便嘱咐其傍晚时分再来。

On the second day, Fei Zhangfang paid respectful tribute to Grandpa Pot with the wine and meat prepared by himself. After knowing Fei Zhangfang's intention, Grandpa Pot felt his sincerity and regarded him as a rough diamond, so he told him to come back in the evening.

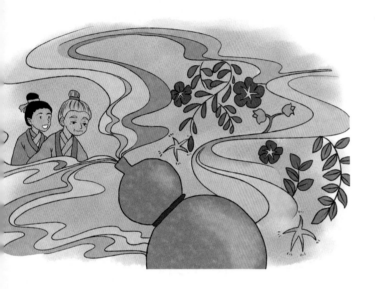

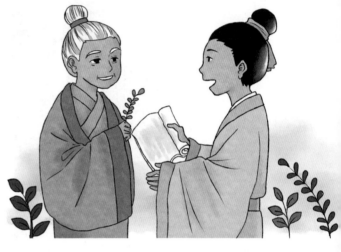

傍晚时分，壶公便邀费长房一起跳入壶中，只见其间处处奇花异草，宛若仙山琼阁。

此后，费长房便拜壶公为师，向他学习医术。

When the time came, Fei Zhangfang was invited to jump with Grandpa Pot into the vessel, inside which an amazing world displayed—fantastic flowers and plants blooming everywhere, just like jade palace of the wonderland.

From then on, Fei Zhangfang worshiped Grandpa Pot as his master, from whom he learned the medical skill.

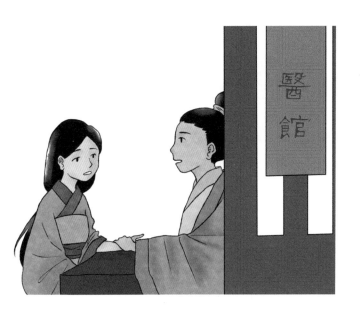

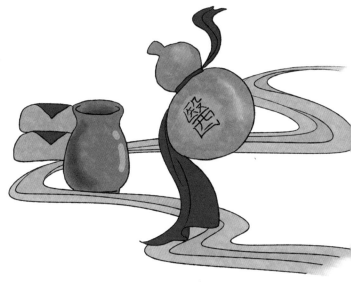

学成之后，费长房返回故里，开始为人疗疾，成了名传千里的医生。

After completing his learning, Fei Zhangfang returned to his hometown and began to work as a doctor, earning his reputation all over China.

古代汉语中"壶"和"葫"同义相通，而这悬壶济世典故中的"壶"便是中药葫芦。为了纪念费长房，葫芦也成了行医的标志，中药的象征。

In ancient Chinese language, "pot" and "gourd" are synonymous, and the "pot" in the story of "hanging pot for the benefit of the world (practicing the medicine to help the people)" is the gourd. To commemorate Fei Zhangfang, people refer to the gourd as the symbol of practicing medicine and traditional Chinese medicine.

葫芦功效
The Efficacy of Gourd

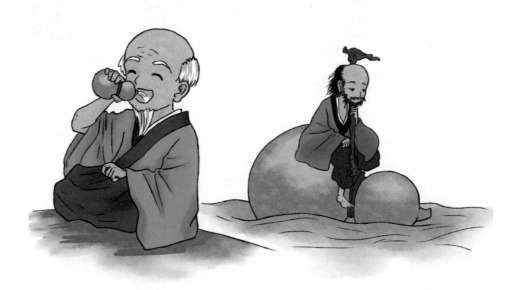

功效分析

无论是医者手中装药盛酒的葫芦，或是八仙过海中有"药王"之称的铁拐李渡海所乘坐的葫芦，都可见葫芦与中医药界相关的元素。不仅如此，葫芦本身亦是一味中药。葫芦味甘性平，最主要的功效是利水消肿，临床可用于心源性水肿、肝硬化腹水等水肿病证的治疗。

Efficacy Analysis

Whether it is the gourd filled with medicine or wine in the hands of doctors or the gourd used by Tie-Guai Li (known as the "King of Medicine" in the legend of *Eight Immortals Crossing the Sea*) to sail across the sea, it can be seen that the gourd is one of the icons related to traditional Chinese medicine. Moreover, the gourd itself is also a traditional Chinese medicine. The gourd has a sweet taste and mild nature. The most important effect of it is to induce water and alleviate edema. Clinically it can be used for treating some edema diseases such as cardiogenic edema, and cirrhosis ascites.

第二部分
巧治顽疾享圣誉

古代医案医话中记载有许多疑难危证，这些病证看似复杂危急，然在医家手中却总能以了了数味药物妙手回春。这其中不仅有医家智慧的荟萃，同时也展现了药与病之间微妙的联结。

Part II
Curing Refractory Illness and Enjoying Holy Reputation

Ancient medical records have documented many difficult, miscellaneous and critical cases, which seemed to be complex and incurable. But in the hands of doctors, these diseases were always able to be treated magically with a few suitable medicines. This embodies not only the crystallization of doctors' great wisdom, but also a delicate relation between medicines and diseases.

智解咽痛
Ginger and Yang Jie

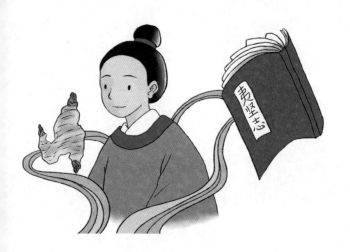

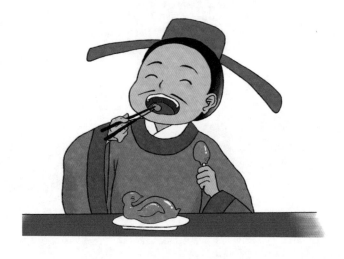

杨介为宋代名医，善治奇病怪病，《夷坚志》中便记载了一则他巧用生姜治喉痛的故事。

据记载宋朝期间，广州通判杨立之喜食一种叫鹧鸪的小鸟。

Yang Jie, a famous doctor in the Song Dynasty, was good at curing some complicated and uncommon diseases. *Tales of Yi Jian*, a collection of ghost stories in the Southern Song Dynasty, records a story about how he treated throat carbuncle by using ginger.

During the Song Dynasty, Yang Lizhi, the prefect of Guangzhou city, enjoyed eating partridges.

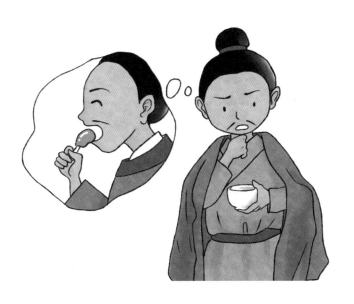

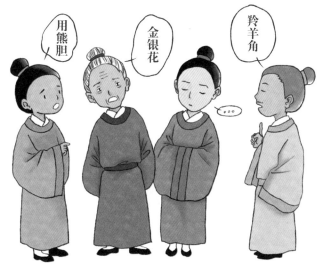

一日吃晚饭，他照例吃了一只鹧鸪。到了临睡前，他突然感到咽痛难忍，连咽口水都很困难，便自行服用了一些清热解毒药。可第二天起床后，却发现咽痛更为严重，肿痛加溃烂，以致寝食难安。

One day he as usual had a partridge for dinner. At bed time, he suddenly felt a sore throat and wasn't able to swallow! Then he took some herbs for clearing heat-toxin on his own, hoping to be better. The next morning, however, he found it even worse—with swollen pain and ulceration, the sore throat made him feel on pins and needles.

他四处寻医，大多数医生都认为是咽喉热毒引起的喉痛，开了大剂量的清热解毒药，但服后都觉无效。

He sought medical advice everywhere. Most doctors believed that throat carbuncle was caused by heat-toxin of throat, and prescribed large doses of herbs for clearing heat-toxin, but none of them worked.

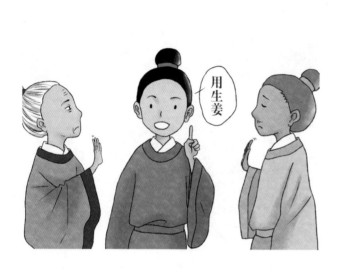

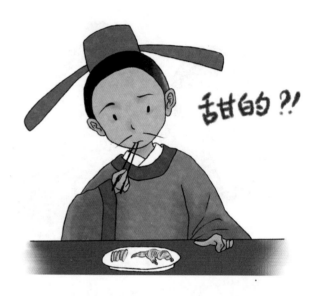

无奈之下，他请来了当时的名医杨介诊治。杨介仔细询问病情后，嘱咐他不应再食用鹧鸪，同时开处一张处方，方中只有一味药："生姜一斤"。众人纷纷摇手，表示不解。

In despair, he invited Yang Jie, a well-known doctor at that time. After carefully inquiring about his condition, Yang Jie told him not to have partridges anymore. Meanwhile, he prescribed a prescription, in which there was only one medicine—"500g of ginger". The crowd doubted, shaking their hands, feeling confused.

抱着将信将疑的态度，杨立之试着吃了两片生姜，奇怪的是他非但不觉得生姜辛辣，反而感觉姜味甘甜。

Though sceptical, Yang Lizhi tried two slices of ginger. Strangely, instead of spicy, he felt a sweet taste of the ginger.

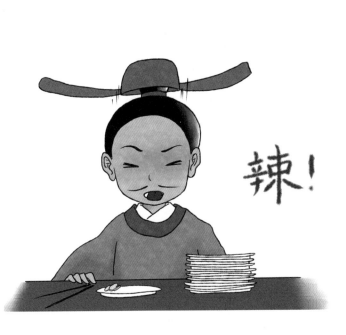

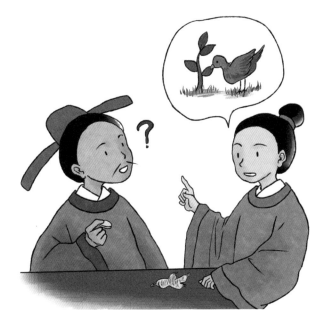

等到吃了"生姜一斤"后，杨立之才逐渐感觉到生姜的辛辣，其咽喉肿痛也已慢慢痊愈。

Having taken 500g of ginger, Yang Lizhi gradually felt spicy of the ginger, and his sore throat had been slowly healed.

欣喜和疑惑间，杨立之向杨介询问其中原委。杨介解释道："这与你所食的鹧鸪有关，鹧鸪喜食生半夏，长久必定中半夏毒，而生姜专解半夏毒，故用生姜治疗才对证。"

Joyful as well as perplexed, Yang Lizhi inquired the doctor. Yan Jie explained, "Your disease is related to the partridges you have taken. Partridges like to eat raw *Pinellia ternata*, and you must have been gradually poisoned by the *Pinellia ternata* from the partridges you have taken. Ginger is a special antidote to *Pinellia ternata*, so it's the only right choice to treat your disease."

生姜功效
The Efficacy of Ginger

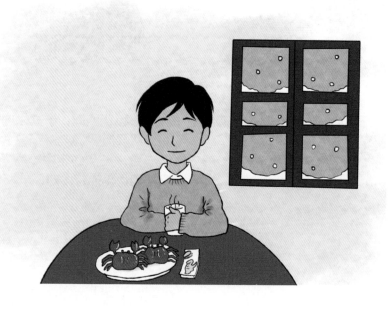

功效分析

故事中的通判喜食鹧鸪，鹧鸪喜食荒山野岭的生半夏，而生半夏有毒，特别是对五官黏膜有刺激。长久食用必中半夏之毒，侵入咽喉而发病。生姜专解半夏之毒，故用生姜治疗才对证。同时生姜还善解食物毒，特别善解鱼蟹之毒，这也是我们吃大闸蟹要蘸姜醋的原因。另外，食用过生姜的人也会感受到其辛辣之味，脸面通红、满头大汗，这与生姜辛辣温散的特性相关。其归于肺胃经，故还具有温散寒邪，温中止呕，温肺止咳的功效。

Efficacy Analysis

In the story, the prefect enjoyed eating partridges, and partridges eat raw *Pinellia ternata* in the wild mountains, which is poisonous and especially stimulates the five senses mucosa. Long-term consumption of *Pinellia ternata* poison invades the throat and develops a disease. The ginger specializes in the detoxification of *Pinellia ternata*, so only ginger can be used to treat for the symptoms. Meanwhile, the ginger is also good at detoxifying food poisoning, especially fish and crab. That is why we eat hairy crabs dipped in ginger vinegar. In addition, people who have eaten ginger will also feel its spicy taste, making faces blushing and sweating, which is related to the characteristics of ginger: spicy and hot in nature. It is classified into the lung and stomach meridians. So it also has the effect of warming and relieving coldness, warming innards and preventing vomiting, warming lung and relieving cough.

巧取内钉
Magnetite and Zhang Jingyue

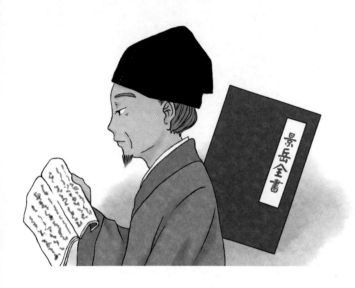

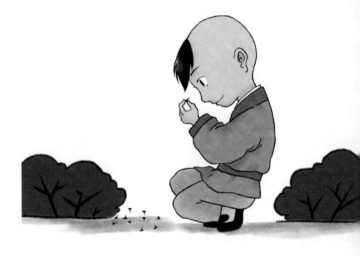

张景岳是明代著名医家，他善用熟地于温补之剂，有"张熟地"之称。不过，如果你认为他只是个慢郎中可就错了，他曾有一段急智解危的故事。

Zhang Jingyue was a well-known doctor in the Ming Dynasty. He was expert in using Shu Di (Radix Rehmanniae) in warming and nourishing prescription, so he was also known as "Zhang Shudi". But don't mistake him as a slow healer. Zhang once won himself some credit with a quick-witted rescue.

一日，一户人家刚满周岁的小孩，在庭院里玩耍。

One day, a one-year-old kid was playing in the courtyard.

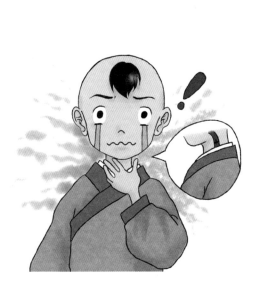

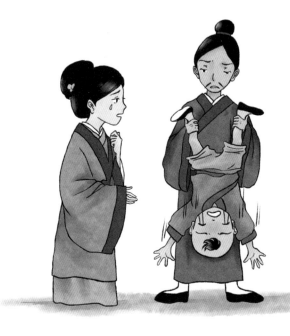

一不小心，小孩将所玩的铁钉误塞入口中，卡在喉间出不来。

By accident, he mistakenly swallowed the nails he was playing with and it got stuck in the throat.

父母见状大惊，忙倒提小孩两足，试图倒出铁钉，但却没用，情况十分危急。

In panic, the parents in no time turned the boy upside down by grabbing his legs, tying to get the nail out, but in vain.

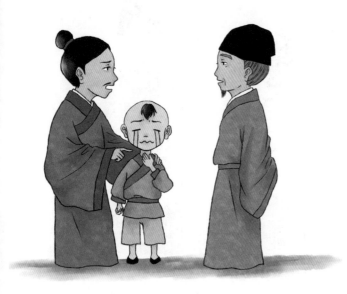

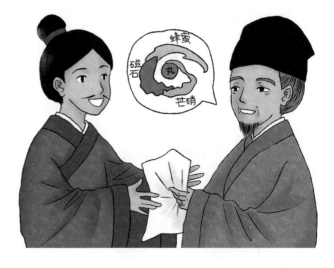

这时恰好张景岳路过，听说了小孩的情况，断定铁钉已入肠胃，小孩父母吓得六神无主，连声哀求张景岳想想办法。

Zhang Jingyue happened to pass by. After hearing about the whole situation, he concluded that the nail must have already reached the stomach. The parents were so frightened that they begged him to save the kid.

张景岳见状沉思片刻，开了三味药：磁石、芒硝、蜂蜜，嘱咐小孩家人将其揉成丸，给小孩服下。

Zhang thought it over for a moment and prescribed three medicines: the magnetite, the mirabilite and the honey. He asked the parents to knead the medicines into a pill for the kid to take.

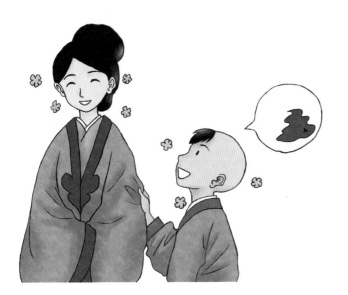

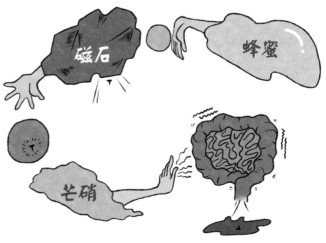

小孩服下后，顿觉腹痛，立马解下一物，其家人拨开一看，里面果有一枚铁钉。

Hardly had he taken the medicine when the kid felt pain in the abdomen and excreted something. His parent poked it open and found there was a nail in it.

小儿父母在感激不尽的同时，向张景岳请教这其中的奥秘。原来磁石具磁性能够吸附铁钉，蜂蜜质滋润可裹护铁钉并保护脾胃，芒硝泻下通便逐铁钉而出，三者共同作用故使危机得解。

The parents felt deeply grateful to Zhang, and Zhang explained the reason to them. The magnetite with the magnetic nature absorbs the iron nail; the honey can wrap the iron nail and protect the spleen and stomach by its moisturizing nature; and the mirabilite has the function of defecation, so combining the functions of these three kinds of medicine, the nail could come out, thus saving the kid's life.

磁石的功效
The Efficacy of Magnetite

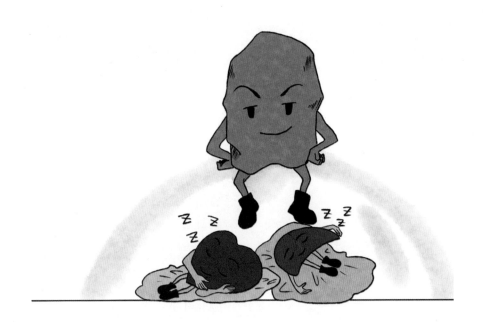

功效分析

磁石质重，具潜降之性，其功效可以归纳为"重镇"二字。一是重镇安神，能够潜降浮越于外的心神，治疗心神不安（类似于失眠）；二是重镇潜阳，能够潜降上亢的肝阳，治疗肝阳上亢引起的眩晕（类似于高血压）。此外，中医理论认为，肾能够使呼吸维持在一定的频率和深度，而磁石的重镇之性还体现在其能够重镇纳气，治疗肾虚气喘。

Efficacy Analysis

The magnetite is heavy and has the potential to submergence, so its efficacy can be summarized as "Zhongzhen (heavy and calm)". Zhongzhen of calming the nerves treats mental disturbance (like insomnia); Zhongzhen of suppressing yang treats vertigo caused by the liver yang hyperactivity (like hypertension). In addition, according to the theory of traditional Chinese medicine, the kidney can maintain breathing at a certain frequency and depth, and the Zhongzhen nature of magnetite is also reflected in its ability to receive qi and treat the dyspnea of kidney deficiency.

起死回生
Squid Bone and Zhu Danxi

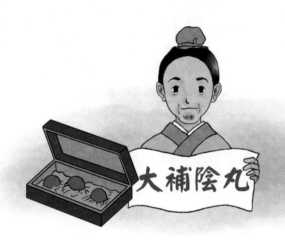

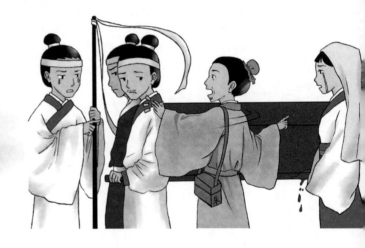

金元时期，医学产生了许多学派，其中朱丹溪善用养阴药物，是滋阴派的代表人物。他还曾留有一段以乌贼骨"起死回生"的传奇故事。

During the Jin Yuan Dynasty, many schools of the medicine science came into being, among which the yin-nourishing school with Zhu Danxi was an outstanding representative good at using yin-nourishing drugs. There was even a story about how he saved the "deceased" by using the squid bones.

一次朱丹溪外出，路遇一队出殡的队列。突然，朱丹溪发现棺材下好像有鲜血滴出，便向家主提出开棺，断定"死者"并没死。

Once Zhu Danxi came across with a funeral procession. Accidentally he noticed some blood dripping from the coffin, so he asked the family to open the coffin, asserting that the one lying inside was not dead.

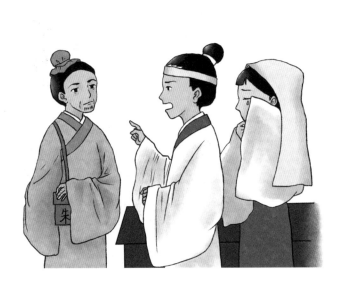

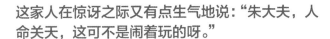

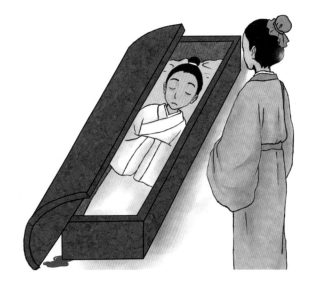

这家人在惊讶之际又有点生气地说："朱大夫，人命关天，这可不是闹着玩的呀。"

Surprised, the family was a little annoyed, saying, "Doctor Zhu, this is a matter of life and death. Please be serious."

朱丹溪态度坚定，"死者"家属也鉴于他是名医，便还是按照他的要求打开了棺材。

Seeing the firmness of the famous doctor, the family finally agreed to open the coffin at his request.

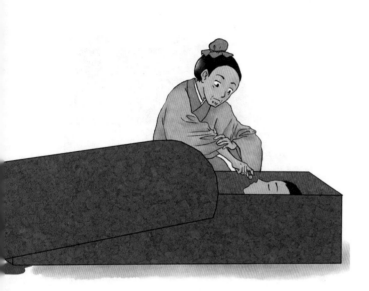

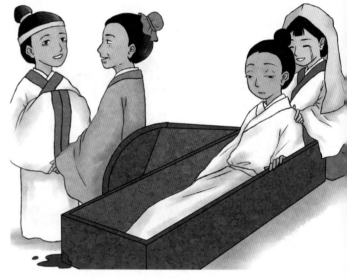

于是朱丹溪上前给"死者"服用了一颗丹药。

Then the doctor made "the dead man" take the pill.

没过多久，"死者"果真醒了过来。"死者"家属百思不解，朱丹溪这才解释道："刚刚我发现棺材还在滴血，而只有活人才会流血，这便断定他并没有死。"

Soon afterwards, "the dead man" woke up. The family were all joyful as well as puzzled, and Zhu Danxi explained, "On seeing the dripping blood from the coffin, I knew immediately that the man was alive, for the dead never bleed."

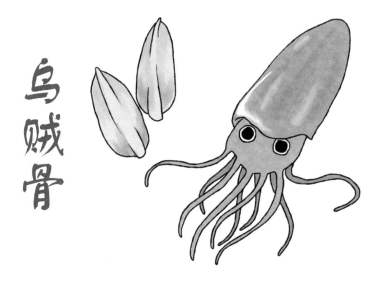

乌贼骨

朱丹溪所用的丸药中其主要成分便是乌贼骨。

The main ingredient of the pill used by Zhu Danxi is
the squid bone.

乌贼骨功效
The Efficacy of Squid Bone

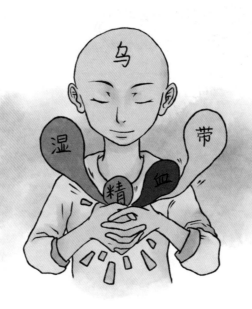

功效分析

故事中的死者只是因为失血量较多而短暂昏迷，并非死亡，而乌贼骨在其中起到了止血的作用。乌贼骨止血与其涩味的特性有关。中医理论中，涩味主收敛固涩，主要用于治疗一些滑脱不禁的病证。乌贼骨为涩味药的代表，其所有的功效都围绕其收涩之性展开，收敛止血，固精止带，制酸止痛，收湿敛疮。

Efficacy Analysis

The patient in the story was only in a temporary coma caused by loss of a large amount of blood, but not truly dead, and the squid bone plays a hemostatic role in it. The squid bone hemostasis is related to its astringent characteristics. In the theory of traditional Chinese medicine, astringency is mainly used to treat some diseases of uncontrollable prostration. The squid bone is a typical astringent medicine. All its effects are centered on the astringency: stanching bleeding, stopping leucorrhea, inhibiting gastric acid and restraining dampness.

第三部分
无心之举显药效

古代医家并非圣人，对药物功效的认识亦须通过长期经验的积累。但他们却善于观察，一些药物的发现便是来源于一些生活中的无心之举。

Part Ⅲ
Inadvertent Action Showing Efficacy

Ancient physicians were not saints, and they came to understand the efficacy of medicines through continuous accumulation of experience. In fact, it was their observant eyes that helped them to discover medicines through common occurrences.

误打误撞
Bezoar and Bian Que

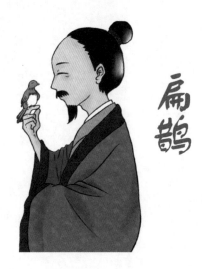

扁鹊

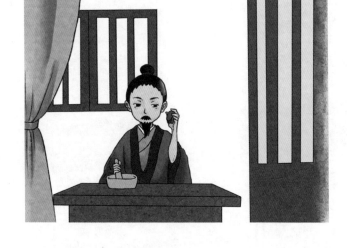

扁鹊原名秦越人，因"灵鹊兆喜"为人带来安康而化名扁鹊，是秦汉时代的名医。相传牛黄这味中药药效的发现便与他有关。

Bian Que, formerly named Qin Yueren, who had this name Que (magpie) after the allusion of "magpie heralding happiness", was a famous doctor in the Qin and Han Dynasties. Legend has it that the discovery of the efficacy of bezoar was credited to him.

一日，扁鹊正研磨青礞石，准备治疗邻居阳文的中风偏瘫之病。

One day, Bian Que was grinding chlorite schist preparing to treat Yang Wen, his neighbor, for his hemiplegia caused by stroke.

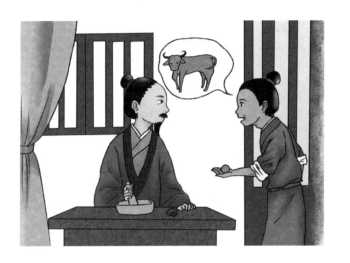

恰逢邻居阳文的儿子阳宝刚杀了一头病牛，却发现牛胆囊中有些像石头样的东西，便来询问。

When Yang Bao, the son of the patient, came for inquiry about something he found in the gallbladder of a sick cattle he had just killed.

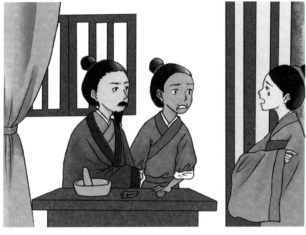
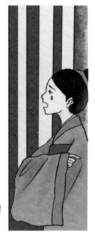

正在这时，阳文的病情突然发作，阳宝便将石头放在桌上，与扁鹊一同前往查看。

Just at that moment, Yang Wen's disease suddenly attacked. On putting the stone-like object on the table, Yang Bao went to see his dad with Bian Que.

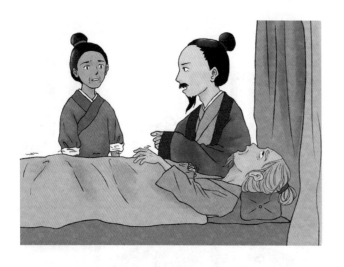

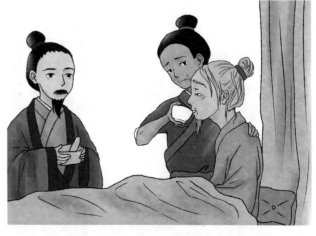

只见阳宝的父亲病眼上视，身体抽搐，喉中痰鸣辘辘，情况十分危急。

The father's eyes rolled back, his body twitching and his throat rumbling with phlegm. The situation was seriously urgent.

扁鹊立即嘱咐阳宝去拿青礞石来。阳宝拿来后，扁鹊未加细察，便将其研为粉末，给病人服下，阳文不一会儿就停止了抽搐，神志也渐渐恢复了。

Immediately Bian Que told Yang Bao to get the chlorite schist. Bian Que, without noticing the "stone" Yang Bao took by mistake, grinded it into powder and helped the patient to take it. After a while, Yang Wen stopped convulsing and gradually recovered his consciousness.

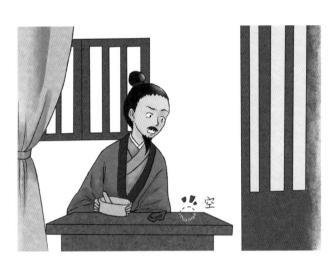

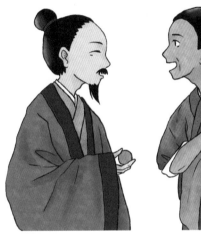

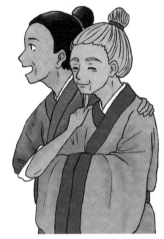

可当扁鹊回到房间查看时，却发现青礞石还在桌上，而牛结石却不见了，这才得知原来阳宝错把牛结石当作青礞石给了自己。

It was not until Bian Que returned to his room that he realized what Yang Bao had given to him was the bezoar not the chlorite schist.

不过，这偶然的差错却使扁鹊意识到这牛结石可能也有豁痰开窍的作用，便有意识地用其为阳文治疗。三日后，阳文的病竟奇迹般好转了。自此以后，牛结石的功用便引起了扁鹊的重视，成了一味治病良药。

However, this accidental incident helped Ban Que have a new understanding of the bezoar: it may also have the effect of expectoration and resuscitation, so he used it continuously for treating Yang Wen. Three days later, Yang Wen's illness was cured miraculously. Since then, the efficacy of bezoar had been carefully studied by Bian Que and was added on the medicine list for treating diseases.

牛黄功效
The Efficacy of Bezoar

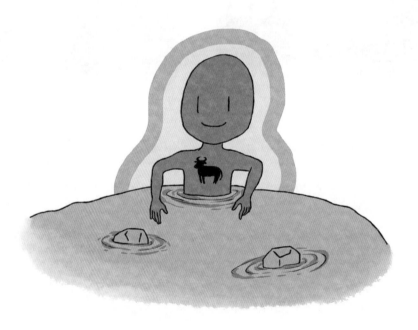

功效分析

牛结石，其色黄，故名牛黄。牛黄久浸于胆汁之中，也被赋予胆汁的特性——味苦而性寒。牛黄归于心、肝经。能够清泻心火而化痰开窍，清泄肝火而息风止痉，同时能够清热解毒。后世医家以牛黄为主药，研制成安宫牛黄丸，对于多种神昏惊厥病证皆用之有效。

Efficacy Analysis

The bezoar, as its color is yellow, is called Niu Huang in Chinese. The bezoar has been immersed in bile for a long time, and the latter endows it with the characteristics of bitter taste and cold nature. The bezoar is also with the channel tropisms in heart and liver. It can clear away the heat of heart and remove phlegm to resuscitate, clear away the liver fire and calm endogenous wind to stop spasm, and at the same time it has the function of clearing away heat-toxin. Later physicians developed "Angong Niuhuang Pill" with the bezoar as the main ingredient, which is effective for many syndromes of coma and convulsion.

因势利导

Veratrum and Zhang Zihe

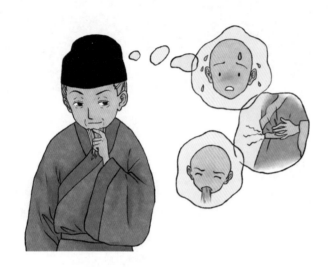

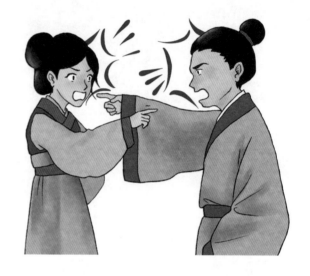

金元四大家中，张子和是攻下派的代表，擅长通过泻下、引吐、发汗的方法祛除病邪，治疗疾病，而其灵感的获得却缘于一段因缘巧合。

Among the four great doctors of the Jin and Yuan Dynasty, Zhang Zihe was the representative of the school of purgation. He was good at curing diseases by means of purgation, induced vomiting and sweating. And his inspiration came from a coincidence.

有一次，张子和的邻居王氏与丈夫大吵了一架后，变得疯疯癫癫、性格暴戾，行事也愈来愈不可理喻。

Once, Wang, Zhang Zihe's neighbor, had a fierce quarrel with her husband, and afterwards she became hysterical, aggressive and unreasonable.

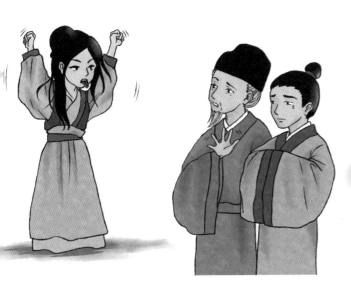

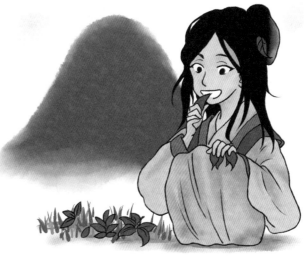

她丈夫恳请张子和为他夫人诊治，但是张看后摇了摇头无奈地说："这病乃是痰入脑窍，病位极深，恐怕非药物可及，我也束手无策。"

Her husband begged Zhang Zihe to treat the wife. But after examining the patient, Zhang shook his head and said helplessly, "This disease is caused by the phlegm entering the brain. The location of disease is so deep inside that I'm afraid it's beyond the reach of drugs. I'm sorry that I can't help with it."

有一天，王氏的疯癫病又突然发作，独自一人跑到了山上拔了许多野草吃。

One day, Wang's disease broke out again. With no reason, she ran to the mountain alone and ate lots of weeds on the slopes.

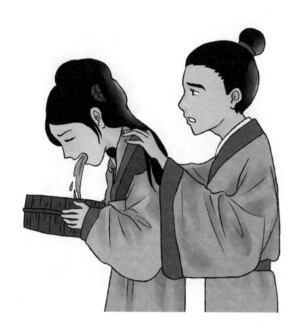

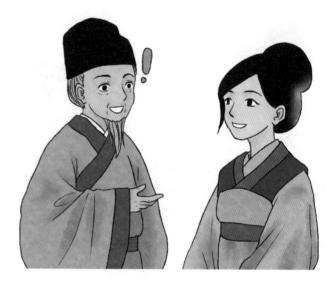

回家后不久，王氏顿觉腹中难受不适，呕吐大作，吐出了许多黏稠如胶的痰涎。

Shortly after returning home, feeling uncomfortable in her abdomen, Wang began to vomit heavily and spit out many sticky sputum and saliva.

不料呕吐完之后，王氏竟然清醒了许多，多年所患的疯癫病竟逐渐好了。张子和见后感到很是疑惑。

Unexpectedly, after vomiting, Wang sobered up a lot, and the illness she had suffered for years gradually improved! Yet, her miraculous recovery very much confused Zhang Zihe.

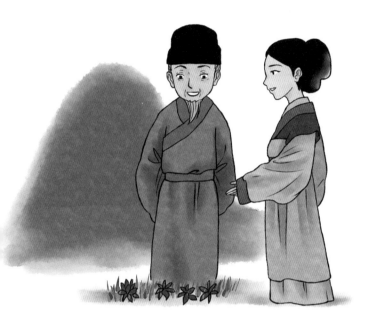

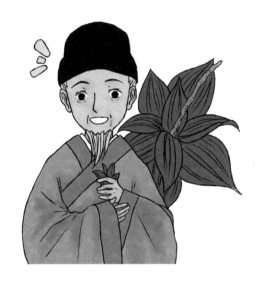

听说了王氏采食野草的经历后，张子和便要求王氏带他去山上，指认了她当时所吃的野草。

Then Zhang asked Wang to take him to identify the weeds she had taken in on the mountains.

张子和见后恍然大悟，这味药便是藜芦，其具有催吐的功效。而利用汗、吐、下等攻邪的方法来治病的思想也逐渐在张子和脑中形成。

The weeds were veratrum plants. Zhang Zihe suddenly realized that the veratrum had the effect of inducing vomiting. The idea of using sweating, vomiting and diarrhea methods to attack pathogens and treat diseases later gradually formed in his mind.

藜芦功效
The Efficacy of Veratrum

藜芦

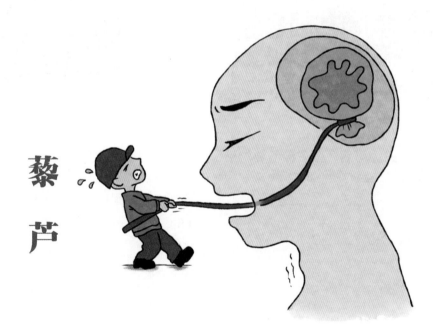

功效分析

藜芦是代表性的涌吐药，对于误食毒物者可以起到类似洗胃的作用。另外，对于故事中王氏的疯癫病，中医认为是风痰上扰脑窍所致，部位相对深邃，较难根除。藜芦催吐作用强烈，可以涌吐风痰，涤痰而出，可用于中风痰壅病证的治疗。

Efficacy Analysis

The veratrum is a typical emetic drug, which plays a similar role in gastric lavage for those who take poisons by mistake. In addition, for Wang's insanity in the story, according to traditional Chinese medicine theory, it was believed to be caused by the phlegm in brain, which is relatively deep and difficult to eradicate. The veratrum has strong emetic effect, which can expel phlegm by inducing vomiting, therefore it can be used for the treatment of stroke syndrome caused by the phlegm.

将错就错

Blighted Wheat and Wang Huaiyin

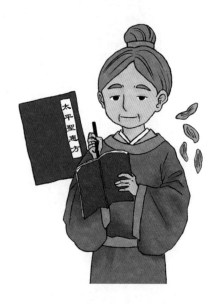

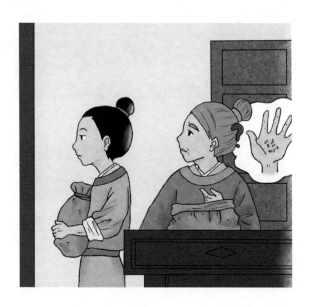

王怀隐是北宋的著名御医，他与陈昭遇等人共同编撰了《太平圣惠方》，也是当时的官修方书。而一次巧合让他发现了浮小麦的作用。

一日，王怀隐发现新购进的小麦又小又瘪，便想询问身边伙计缘由。然而这时，外面却忽然送来了一个病人。

Wang Huaiyin was a famous imperial doctor in the Northern Song Dynasty. He and Chen Zhaoyu co-authored *Taiping Holy and Benevolent Prescription*, an officially-revised book at that time. A coincidence led him to discover the efficacy of the blighted wheat.

One day, Wang Huaiyin found that the newly purchased wheat was neither big nor plump, and just as he was about to ask his lads, however, a patient was suddenly sent in.

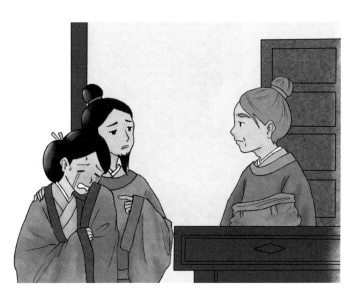

病人丈夫焦急地对王怀隐道："我夫人近来时常发怒，哭笑无常，还时常出汗，湿透衣襟，是不是得了什么重病？"

The patient's husband anxiously said to Wang Huaiyin, "Recently my wife is often ill-tempered and appears cry laugh fugacious. Plus she sweats a lot, soaking up her skirts. Is she suffering from any serious disease?"

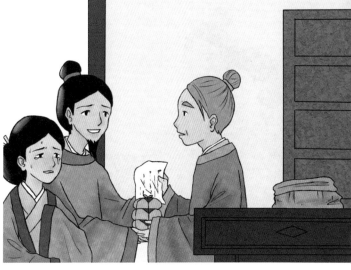

王怀隐看后说道："你不必焦急，这是脏躁病，并不难治。"于是，便开了一个处方：甘草、小麦、大枣。之后，他又补充道："出汗与脏躁并无关系，暂且等其痊愈后再作治疗。"

After examining the wife, Wang Huaiyin told the husband, "You don't need to worry. It's the hysteria, quite common and curable." So he wrote a prescription: licorice, wheat and dates. "Sweating has nothing to do with hysteria, so wait till hysteria is treated," he added.

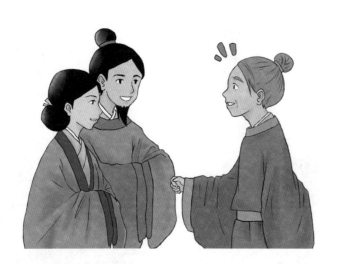

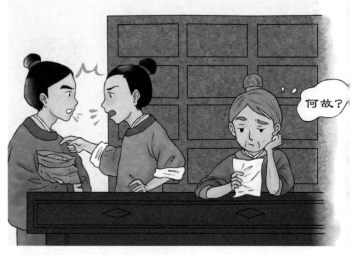

五日后，病人痊愈，前来拜谢，王怀隐诧异地发现，她的出汗症竟也一并好了。他暗自思忖：难道此方也有止汗的作用？

Five days later, the patient recovered and came to thank him. Wang Huaiyin was surprised to find that her sweating disorder had also been cured. He thought to himself, does this prescription also help antiperspiration?

于是他便有意识地以此方治疗几个出汗的病人，但却均不见效。这时伙计的争执声又一次惊动了王怀隐，原来这次收来的小麦也是又小又瘪的。

So he intentionally used this prescription to treat several sweating patients, but in vain. At this very moment, the quarrel of his lads aroused Wang Huaiyin's attention. The wheat purchased this time again was small, flesh thin and looked withered.

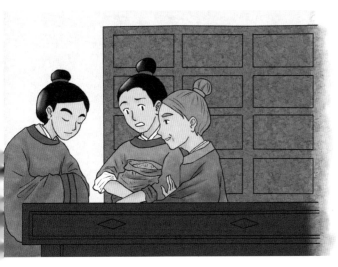

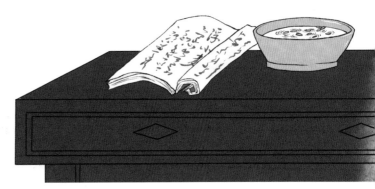

王怀隐听罢，忆起了上次那妇人用的正是这种小麦，似乎悟出了什么，便嘱咐伙计先收下。由于这些麦子能够漂浮于水面，便注明其为浮小麦。

While listening, Wang suddenly recalled that it was this kind of wheat that he treated the woman with. It seemed as if he had understood something, so he asked the lad to take the wheat. Since this kind of wheat could float on the surface of the water, it was identified as "Fu (floating) wheat".

后来，王怀隐用浮小麦试治出汗病证，逐渐认识到浮小麦止汗的功效，并将其功效记录在了《太平圣惠方》一书中。

Later, Wang Huaiyin tried to cure sweating disease with blighted wheat. He gradually realized the anti-perspiration effect of blighted wheat and recorded it in the book *Taiping Holy and Benevolent Prescription*.

浮小麦功效
The Efficacy of Blighted Wheat

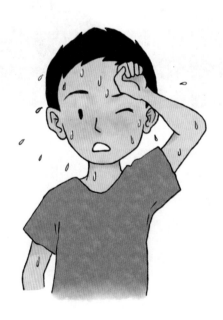

功效分析

浮小麦为小麦干瘪轻浮的颖果，是出汗的对症用药，一切出汗病证都可以用浮小麦来止汗。故事中王怀隐用于治疗脏躁病所用的小麦为淮小麦，是小麦的成熟颖果，能够补益心气、滋养心阴，用于心神不安、妇人脏躁等。

Efficacy Analysis

The blighted wheat is a dry and light caryopsis of wheat. It is a symptomatic drug for sweating. It can be used to prevent all sweating diseases and syndromes. In the story, the wheat used by Wang Huaiyin to treat hysteria is Huai wheat, which is the mature caryopsis of wheat. It can nourish the heart-qi as well as heart-yin, and help to treat restlessness and hysteria of women.

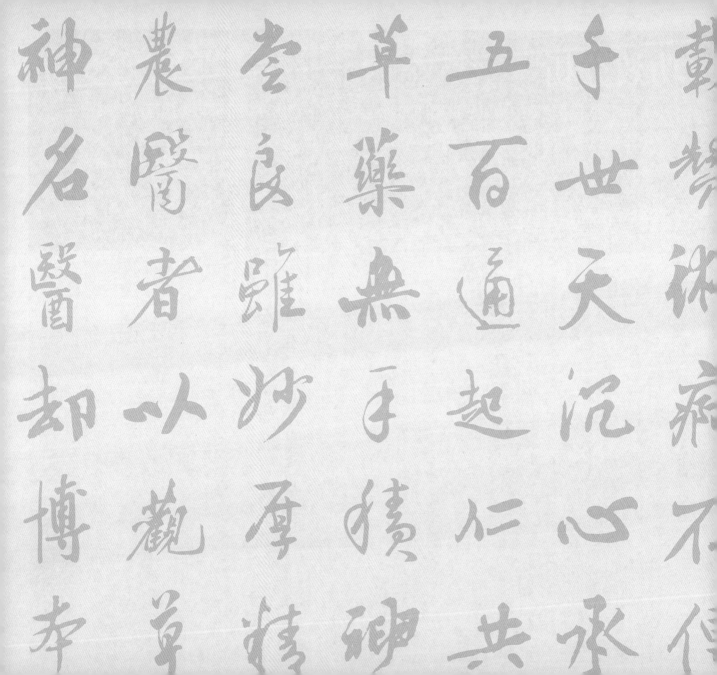